Liver
Rescue

Diet

Cookbook

Recipes that will help you sleep well, balance blood sugar, lower blood pressure, lose weight, and look and feel younger.

By

Emily W. Jones

Copyright page

Copy write @ 2019 by Emily W. Jones

Printed in the U.S.A

Table of Contents

INTRODUCTION:...6

Liver Rescue and How to Redeem the Situation......................6

The following lifestyle changes can help remedy and even
reverse your liver problem...6

The Liver Rescue Recipes 9

Chicken and Grape Salad 9

Raspberry Chia Pudding 11

Grain Free Egg Muffins...13

Roast Pumpkin And Quinoa Salad.......................................14

Avocado And Tomato Salad 16

Chocolate And Hazelnut Fudge...18

Salmon Patties 19

Cleansing Green Juice 21

Low Carb Crackers..22

Sugar Free Tangy Salad Dressing 24

Cinnamon Protein Balls..25

Dairy Free Chocolate Pudding...26

Low FODMAP Tuna Salad..27

Vegan Chickpea And Pumpkin Salad....................................28

Tender Thyme Lamb Cutlets 30

Dairy Free Warming Parsnip Soup 32

Shrimp And Broccoli Stir Fry 34

Nourishing Chicken Soup 36

Gluten Free Gingerbread Protein Balls 38

Bowel Cleansing Smoothie...40

Coffee Cacao Porridge 41

Avocado And Tuna Salad..42

Dairy Free Cranberry Chocolate Bark 43

Gluten and Dairy Free Peanut Butter Banana Cake..............45

Gluten And Dairy Free Peanut Butter Banana Cake 47

Oven Baked Omelette..49

Cacao And Almond Smoothie Bowl 51

Coconut Seafood Curry 52

Gallbladder Cleansing Juice 54

Garlic Spicy Chicken 55

Sugar Free Coconut Balls 56

Vegetarian Quinoa Pilaf 57

Tuna Steaks with Avocado 59

Walnut Basil Pesto 61

Cumin Roasted Macadamia Nuts...62

Garlic Bok Choy Stir Fry..63

Easy Lemon Baked Salmon 64

One Pan Chicken Dinner 65

Low Carb Salmon Salad 67

Grilled Garlic Chicken..68

Detoxifying Green Smoothie 69

Garlic Roasted Broccoli 70

Greek Yogurt and Cucumber Dip 71

Clean Green Smoothie 72

Grain and Dairy Free Almond Breakfast Pancakes 73

Grain Free Bircher-Style Muesli 75

Creamy Cantaloupe Smoothie 76

Nut Free Bliss Balls 77

Dairy Free Creamy Lemon Sauce 78

Refreshing Watermelon Smoothie 79

Date and Tahini Fudge 80

Balsamic Roasted Tomatoes 82

Tender Grilled Baby Octopus 83

Mediterranean Beef Skewers 85

Chicken And Orange Salad 87

Sugar Free Banana Oat Bars 88

Choc Mint Protein Smoothie 89

Pumpkin and Pecan Casserole 90

Kidney Cleansing Juice 92

Chunky Avocado Salsa 93

Conclusion 94

INTRODUCTION:
Liver Rescue and How to Redeem the Situation

Record has it that fatty liver disease affects nearly 1/3 of American adults and is one of the leading contributors to liver failure. Nonalcoholic fatty liver disease is common among people who are obese or sedentary and those who eat a highly processed diet.

These days we probably don't give much thought to our liver (except when you contemplate that third vodka soda), but its health is key to your overall health and weight. However, your liver is the ultimate multitasker: It acts as a filter to dispose toxins (like medications and alcohol from the body) and nutrient byproducts such as it helps in digestion by producing bile to aid in breaking down fat and absorbing fat- and water-soluble vitamins and minerals; ammonia from the blood; and it plays a major part in regulating glucose, blood sugar, estrogen, immunity, blood pressure, insulin, testosterone, and blood cholesterol production and removal. And you thought you had a long to-do list, certainly you must be kidding!

Your liver may be in need of a little TLC because of all the activities it does. When your liver is overworked, toxic residues can build up, causing inflammation that is associated with obesity. A stressed out liver has the tendency to build up fat, especially around the belly. This can mean one thing; that no matter how much you restrict calories; weight loss is near impossible—unless you detox your liver.

The following lifestyle changes can help remedy and even reverse your liver problem.

1. You are advice to adhere to the following lifestyle if you want to help remedy or reverse your liver problems:

2. Stop smoking and use medications only when necessary, as even taking a Tylenol can have severe consequences on the liver.
3. Consumption of alcohol is not good for the liver
4. Generally, you are advice to eat and drink clean. Foods and beverages that contain high-fructose corn syrup, hydrogenated oils, additives, hormones, preservatives, or artificial colors, are harmful to the liver and eat free-range or organic whenever possible. Remember, your liver has to work harder to filter all this gunk.
5. I suggest you consume more of cruciferous vegetables such as broccoli, cauliflower, collards, Brussels sprouts, kale, and cabbage. This is because such contain Sulphur compounds called glucosinolates that bind and eliminate toxins.
6. Abstain from salt, which can contribute to fluid retention and further strain the liver, and flavor foods with rosemary, garlic, dandelion, or chicory, which appear to support liver function.
7. Regular exercise the same way you take your prescription medicine. Your target should be at least a half hour, though more can be better, and be sure you're doing intervals, which will help melt fat. A review published in the Journal of Herpetology found that a combination of diet and exercise daily contributes to the reduction of body weight and therefore improve liver health.
8. Abstain from sugary foods such as cookies, candy, sodas, and fruit juices. High blood sugar increases the amount of fat buildup in the liver.
9. Consumption of coffee to reduce the effect of abnormal liver enzymes. People with fatty liver disease who love drinking coffee experience less liver damage than those who do not drink caffeinated beverage. This is because

caffeine minimizes the risk of abnormal liver enzymes in individuals in high risk of liver disease

10. Anti-inflammatory and fat lowering effect of fish such as sardines, salmon, tuna, and trout which are fatty fish contains high quantity of omega-3 fatty acids. Omega-3 fatty acids can help improve liver fat levels and bring down inflammation. I will suggest you try teriyaki halibut recipe, recommended by the Canadian Liver Foundation, that's especially low in fat.

11. Carbohydrates food from whole grains like oatmeal give your body energy. Their fiber content also fills you up, which can help you maintain your weight.

12. Avocados are high in healthy fats and helps to protect the liver, and research suggests they contain chemicals that might slow liver damage. Nevertheless, they're also rich in fiber, which can help with weight control.

13. Dairy like milk and other low-fat dairy protect the liver from damage. It is high in whey protein, which may protect the liver from further damage.

The Liver Rescue Recipes

Chicken and Grape Salad

A tasty recipe using leftover cooked chicken.

Serves 4

Ingredients:

2 hard-boiled eggs (sliced)

2 stalks of celery (sliced)

Flesh from 1 avocado (sliced)

2 tablespoons of olive oil and (preferably 2 tablespoons of lemon juice, as dressing)

1lb leftover chicken (cooked)

1 cup of red or preferably green grapes (sliced in half or leave whole)

½ cup of chopped toasted pecans

2 large ripe tomatoes (diced)

Directions:

1. **First, you p**lace all salad ingredients into a bowl and mix gently.

2. **Then you,** drizzle with oil and lemon juice, toss gently and serve.

Raspberry Chia Pudding

This recipe is delicious and filling breakfast that's particularly nice on a hot summer morning.

Serves 2

Ingredients

1 cup of coconut milk

2 tablespoons of plain full fat yogurt

2 tablespoon of flaked almonds

1 cup of fresh (or preferably frozen raspberries)

3 tablespoons of chia seeds

A few drops of liquid stevia (to taste)

Directions:

1. First, you process all of the ingredients except the chia seeds and almonds in a food processor or blender until smooth.
2. After which you stir in the chia seeds and divide mixture into two bowls.

3. Then, after 5 minutes stir the mixture again and then place in the fridge overnight.
4. Finally, the next morning sprinkle with flaked almonds and enjoy for breakfast.

Grain Free Egg Muffins

These recipe is high in protein and great for breakfast on the run.

Ingredients

¼ red onion (finely diced)

1 handful parsley (finely chopped)

1 tablespoon of pesto

6 large eggs (whisked)

3 oz. of pastured bacon (finely chopped)

½ red pepper (preferably capsicum), finely diced

Directions:

1. Meanwhile, you heat oven to 350 degrees F.
2. After which you whisk the eggs with the pesto until well combined.
3. After that, you stir in remaining ingredients.
4. At this point, you pour mix into greased muffin tins and bake for approximately 20 minutes, or until golden brown.
5. Finally, baking time will depend on the size of your muffin tins.

Roast Pumpkin and Quinoa Salad

Note: serves 4 as a side salad

Ingredients

1 tablespoon of olive oil

½ teaspoon of ground coriander

2 cups of cooked quinoa

¼ cup of toasted pine nuts

Additional drizzle of olive oil (preferably for dressing)

1-pound pumpkin (peeled and chopped into bite sized pieces)

1 teaspoon of ground cumin

½ teaspoon of salt

¼ cup of fresh parsley (chopped)

2 tablespoons of lemon juice

Directions:

1. First, you place the pumpkin on a lined baking tray.
2. After which you sprinkle with salt, cumin and coriander, then drizzle with olive oil.

3. After that, you roast the pumpkin in the oven until soft and lightly browned.
4. Then, once cool, combine all ingredients in a serving bowl except the lemon juice and additional olive oil; toss gently.
5. Finally, you drizzle with lemon juice and olive oil and serve.

Avocado and Tomato Salad

Make sure you serve it with some protein such as chicken or fish.

Serves 2

Ingredients

1 cup of cherry or preferably grape tomatoes, halved

2 stalks celery (sliced)

¼ red onion (sliced finely)

1 large avocado (diced)

1 handful of basil leaves (torn)

1 small cucumber (sliced)

Dressing ingredients

4 tablespoons of lemon juice

Herb Amare, or salt and spices (to taste)

4 tablespoons of avocado oil (or preferably olive oil)

Directions:

1. First, you combine all salad ingredients together in a bowl.

2. After which you whisk dressing ingredients together well in a small bowl and then pour over salad.
3. Finally, you serve.

Chocolate and Hazelnut Fudge

Ingredients

2 tablespoons of full fat canned coconut cream

¼ cup of chopped roasted hazelnuts

7 ounces of dark chocolate (preferably 85 or 90% cocoa)

Directions:

1. First, you melt the chocolate and coconut cream together.
2. After which you stir until smooth.
3. After that, you stir in hazelnuts and pour mixture into mini muffin patties.
4. Then you place in the fridge to set.

Salmon Patties

Ingredients

1 large sweet potato (cooked and mashed)

½ red onion (finely diced)

1 tablespoon of lemon juice

Salt and pepper (to taste)

2 x 14 ounce of cans salmon (drained)

2/3 cup of almond meal

2 tablespoons of parsley (finely chopped)

2 eggs

Directions:

1. First, you place all ingredients into a large bowl and mix thoroughly with your hands. (**NOTE:** if the mixture is too dry, I suggest you add a little water or more lemon juice. Secondly, if it is too wet, add more almond meal).
2. Remember, this will depend on the moisture content of the sweet potato you're using.
3. After which you form the mixture into patties.

NOTE: you can either bake them on a lined oven tray or fry them on a pan in ghee, olive oil or coconut oil.

4. Then you bake for about 20 minutes at 355 degrees F.
5. Finally, you serve with a salad.

Cleansing Green Juice

Serves 1

Ingredients

1 stalk of celery

1 green apple

1 Lebanese cucumber

1 lime (peeled if not organic)

Directions:

1. First, you pass all ingredients through a juice extractor and drink.

Low Carb Crackers

It makes approximately 20 crackers

Ingredients

1 large egg (whisked)

1 teaspoon of dried oregano

2 cups of blanched almond flour

½ teaspoon of salt

Directions:

1. Meanwhile, you heat the oven to 350 degrees F.
2. After which you mix all ingredients together well in a bowl, and then use your hands to mix everything together and create a dough.
3. After that, you place the dough between two sheets of parchment paper.
4. Then you roll it out until it's thin and to your liking.
5. At this point, you remove the top sheet of parchment paper, and place the bottom sheet, with the dough onto a baking tray.

6. This is when you mark the dough into cracker sized pieces with a knife or pizza cutter.
7. Finally, you bake in the oven for approximately 10 to 15 minutes, or until lightly browned and cooked through.
8. Make sure you allow to cool and then serve.

Sugar Free Tangy Salad Dressing

Makes ¾ cup

Ingredients

1 clove garlic (crushed)

½ teaspoon of salt

2 tablespoons of finely chopped fresh parsley

¾ cup of plain full fat Greek yogurt

2 tablespoons of finely chopped fresh chives or preferably spring onion

2 tablespoons of lemon juice

1 teaspoon of Dijon mustard

Directions:

1. First, you place the ingredients into a blender and blend until combined, or preferably, you whisk them together well in a bowl.

Cinnamon Protein Balls

Ingredients

1 cup of unsweetened shredded coconut

2 tablespoons of almond butter

1 teaspoon of ground cinnamon

Approximately 4 tablespoons of almond milk

1 cup of almond meal

1 tablespoon of Synd-X Slimming whey protein powder

5 Medjool dates (pits removed)

1 teaspoon of vanilla extract

Directions:

1. First, you place all ingredients into a food processor and process until smooth.
2. Remember, the amount of almond milk necessary will vary and depends on the moisture content of the dates and shredded coconut you use.
3. Finally, you shape the mixture into balls and store in an airtight container in the fridge.

Dairy Free Chocolate Pudding

Serves 2

Ingredients

¼ cup of cacao or preferably cocoa powder (sifted)

1 teaspoon of vanilla extract

¾ cup of canned full fat coconut cream

2 tablespoons of maple syrup or preferably honey

1 tablespoon of chia seeds

Directions:

1. First, you combine all ingredients in a saucepan over medium heat.
2. Remember, that stirring the whole time, bring the mixture to a gentle simmer.
3. After which you cook for a few minutes, until the mixture thickens.

NOTE: you can pour the mixture into serving bowls and chill in the fridge overnight, or preferably enjoy it hot.

Low FODMAP Tuna Salad

Ingredients

1 small zucchini (grated coarsely)

½ Lebanese cucumber (sliced)

6 oz. canned tuna (drained)

1 tablespoon of lemon juice

1 handful of arugula leaves

½ cup of cherry tomatoes (halved)

½ teaspoon of dried oregano

2 tablespoons of olive oil

Directions:

1. First, you mix all salad ingredients together gently.
2. Then you drizzle with olive oil and lemon juice.

Vegan Chickpea and Pumpkin Salad

Serves 4

Ingredients

2 tablespoons of olive oil

1 teaspoon of ground coriander

1 small red onion (thinly sliced)

1 handful of parsley (chopped)

Salt and pepper (to taste)

1 cup of peeled and diced pumpkin (preferably chopped into bite sized pieces)

1 teaspoon of ground cumin

1 (15oz) can chickpeas (rinsed and drained)

1 avocado (diced)

1 tablespoon of lemon juice

Directions:

1. Meanwhile, you roast the pumpkin.
2. After which you arrange it on a lined oven tray, drizzle with olive oil and sprinkle with cumin and coriander.
3. After that, you roast until the pumpkin is soft and lightly browned.

4. Then you arrange all salad ingredients together in a bowl.
5. Finally, you drizzle with lemon juice and serve.

Tender Thyme Lamb Cutlets

This recipe is a quick and tasty low carb recipe that will please the whole family.

Serves 4

Ingredients

2 tablespoons of dried thyme

Salt and pepper (to taste)

12 lamb cutlets

4 tablespoons of fresh lemon juice

4 tablespoons of olive oil

Directions:

1. First, you place the cutlets into a glass bowl.
2. After which you drizzle the lemon juice and olive oil on top, and using your hands, make sure each cutlet is well coated.
3. Then you cover the bowl and place in the fridge overnight.

4. After that, you place the cutlets on a grill or barbecue and sprinkle with salt, thyme, and pepper.
5. At this point, you cook for about 2 to 3 minutes on each side.
6. Finally, you serve with roasted or steamed vegetables.

Dairy Free Warming Parsnip Soup

This recipe is thick and hearty, without the cream to weigh down your liver and it is delicious served as an appetizer.

Serves 4

Ingredients

1 brown onion (finely chopped)

2 medium carrots (chopped)

½ cup of chopped pumpkin

1 tablespoon of dried oregano

Salt and pepper (to taste)

1 tablespoon of olive oil

3 garlic cloves (crushed)

4 medium parsnips (chopped)

5 cups of stock or preferably broth

1 teaspoon of ground cumin

Directions:

1. First, you heat the oil in a large pot over medium heat.
2. After which you sauté the garlic and onion until slightly softened.
3. After that, you stir in all remaining ingredients except the broth or stock.
4. Then you cook, stirring for about 2 minutes.
5. At this point, you add broth or stock, bring the mixture to the boil and then reduce heat and simmer until all the vegetables are soft.
6. Finally, you puree the soup and serve.

Shrimp and Broccoli Stir Fry

Serves 2

Ingredients

1 large handful of roasted cashews

3 tablespoons of coconut aminos

2 cloves garlic (crushed)

2 tablespoons of lime juice

Salt and pepper (to taste)

1 head broccoli (make sure you cut into small florets and lightly steamed)

2 tablespoons of macadamia nut oil (remember to duck fat or olive oil)

1 tablespoon of fish sauce

½ red pepper (preferably capsicum), sliced

8 oz. shrimp (peeled)

1 tablespoon of sesame seeds

Directions:

1. First, you heat the oil or duck fat in a frying pan or wok.

2. After which you add the red pepper, garlic, sesame seeds and cashews.
3. After that, you add the shrimp and stir fry for a few minutes, until they are almost cooked.
4. Then you add broccoli.
5. At this point, you whisk lime juice, salt, coconut aminos, fish sauce, and pepper together in a bowl.
6. Finally, you pour mixture into frying pan and cook.

Nourishing Chicken Soup

Serves 4

NOTE: this soup uses leftover cooked chicken.

This recipe is quick and simple to prepare, while being easily digested and gentle on your gut.

Ingredients

1 cup of canned coconut cream

2 tablespoons of olive oil

1 large zucchini (sliced)

2 stalks celery (sliced)

2 bay leaves

Salt and pepper (to taste)

5 cups of bone broth, or preferably stock

4 cups of cooked, shredded chicken

2 large carrots (diced)

1 small brown onion (diced)

1 medium swede or better still turnip (diced)

2 teaspoons of dried oregano

Directions:

1. First, you sauté all of the vegetables in the olive oil, in a large pot until the onion has softened.
2. After which you add all remaining ingredients except the coconut cream.
3. After that, once the vegetables have softened to your liking, add the coconut cream, stir through well.
4. Finally, you take off the heat, garnish with parsley and serve.

Gluten Free Gingerbread Protein Balls

This is a delicious, festive recipe that will enable you to still fit into your jeans this holiday season.

Ingredients

1 cup of roasted almonds

1 tablespoon of ground ginger

2 tablespoons of honey or preferably 1 teaspoon of Nature Sweet

1 cup of roasted walnuts

½ cup of unsweetened desiccated coconut

1 teaspoon of ground cloves

1 tablespoon of chia seeds

Directions:

1. First, you place all ingredients into a food processor and blend until ground and the mixture comes together.

NOTE: if the mixture is a little dry, I suggest you add a little water.

2. Finally, you form mixture into balls and store in an airtight container in the fridge.

Bowel Cleansing Smoothie

This fiber-rich smoothie recipe will help to keep your colon clean and flatten out a bloated belly.

Serves 1

Ingredients

1 tablespoon of Fiber tone

1 banana

1 ½ cups of nut or preferably seed milk of your choice

1 tablespoon of almond butter

2 tablespoons of Synd-X whey protein powder

Directions:

1. First, you place all ingredients into a blender.
2. Then you blend until smooth.

Coffee Cacao Porridge

Serves 1

Ingredients

¼ cup of brewed coffee

½ cup of rolled oats

¼ cup of chopped (roasted pecans)

1 tablespoon of cacao powder

1 teaspoon of vanilla extract

¾ cup of hemp or preferably almond milk

Directions:

1. First, you place all ingredients except pecans and vanilla into a small pot and cook gently over medium heat.
2. After which you stir regularly and add a little more milk if the mixture becomes too thick.
3. After that, you cook until the oats have softened to your liking.
4. Then you stir in the vanilla and pecans and enjoy.

Avocado and Tuna Salad

This recipe is a quick, easy and delicious low carb lunch that will leave you feeling satisfied for hours.

Serves 1

Ingredients

½ cup of cherry tomatoes (sliced in half)

½ medium avocado (diced)

5 oz. canned tuna in brine (drained and flaked)

2 tablespoons of olive oil

1 large handful of arugula leaves

½ Lebanese cucumber (sliced)

2 tablespoons of hemp seeds

1 tablespoon of fresh lemon or preferably lime juice

Direction:

1. First, you combine all salad ingredients in a bowl.
2. Then you drizzle with lemon or lime juice and olive oil.

Dairy Free Cranberry Chocolate Bark

This antioxidant-rich dessert recipe is made of whole foods.

NOTE: the healthy fats in coconut oil help to fuel your metabolism.

Ingredients

½ cup of melted coconut oil

¼ cup of dried cranberries

Generous pinch of sea salt

½ cup of cacao (or preferably cocoa powder)

¼ cup of honey (melted)

¼ cup of roasted pecan pieces

Directions:

1. First, you mix the first 3 ingredients together well in a bowl.
2. After which you pour the mixture onto a baking tray that has been lined with baking paper or foil.
3. After that, you smooth it out evenly.
4. Then you sprinkle remaining ingredients evenly over the chocolate mixture.

5. At this point, you place the tray into the freezer to set for about 30 minutes.
6. Finally, you break the bark up and store in an airtight container in the fridge.

Gluten and Dairy Free Peanut Butter Banana Cake

Ingredients

4 eggs (whisked)

4 tablespoons of softened coconut oil

¼ cup of chopped pecans

1 teaspoon of cinnamon

1 teaspoon of baking powder

4 very ripe bananas (mashed)

½ cup of peanut butter

½ cup of almond meal

1 teaspoon of ground cloves

1 teaspoon of baking soda

Directions:

1. Meanwhile, you heat the oven to 350 degrees F.
2. After which you combine the eggs, mashed bananas, and peanut butter in a blender or food processor.
3. After that, you process until smooth.

4. Then you combine all ingredients in a bowl and mix well by hand until combined.
5. At this point, you pour mixture into greased cake tin and bake for approximately one hour, or until an inserted toothpick comes out clean.
6. Finally, you store the cake in an airtight container in the fridge.

Gluten and Dairy Free Peanut Butter Banana Cake

Ingredients

4 eggs (whisked)

4 tablespoons coconut oil (softened)

¼ cup of chopped pecans

1 teaspoon of cinnamon

1 teaspoon of baking powder

4 very ripe bananas (mashed)

½ cup of peanut butter

½ cup of almond meal

1 teaspoon of ground cloves

1 teaspoon of baking soda

Directions:

1. Meanwhile, you heat the oven to 350 degrees F.
2. After which you combine the mashed bananas, eggs and peanut butter in a blender or food processor.

3. After that, you process until smooth.
4. Then you combine all ingredients in a bowl and mix well by hand until combined.
5. At this point, you pour mixture into greased cake tin and bake for approximately one hour, or until an inserted toothpick comes out clean.
6. Finally, you store the cake in an airtight container in the fridge.

Oven Baked Omelets

Serves 4

Ingredients

1 tablespoon of olive oil or preferably other cooking fat

1 large red pepper (preferably capsicum), chopped

¼ cup of olives (sliced in half)

1 teaspoon of dried oregano

8 eggs

1 cup of finely chopped pumpkin

1 red onion (diced)

1/3 cup of full fat coconut milk

1/3 cup of chopped, cooked pastured bacon (it is optional)

Directions:

1. Meanwhile, you heat the oven to 400 degrees F.

2. After which you sauté the onion and pumpkin in the olive oil, over medium heat until fragrant and lightly softened.
3. After that, you add the pepper.
4. Then you cook for another few minutes.
5. At this point, you whisk the eggs with the milk in a large bowl.
6. Furthermore, you arrange all ingredients in a large baking dish and pour egg mixture on top.
7. Finally, you bake for approximately 30 minutes; serve.

Cacao and Almond Smoothie Bowl

Serves 1

With this rich, creamy smoothie bowl you'll feel like you're eating dessert for breakfast.

Ingredients

1 cup of coconut milk

1 heaped of tablespoon almond butter

Flaked almonds

1 frozen sliced banana

1 heaped tablespoon of cacao powder

2 tablespoons of whey protein powder

1 tablespoon of chia seeds

Directions:

1. First, you place all ingredients except flaked almonds into a blender and blend until smooth.
2. Then you pour into bowl and sprinkle flaked almonds on top.
3. Enjoy

Coconut Seafood Curry

Serves 2

Ingredients

One (13 ½ oz.) can full fat coconut milk

2 large carrots (chopped)

1 cup of diced pumpkin

2 tablespoons of curry powder

1 teaspoon of freshly grated ginger

1 lb. of white fresh fish of your choice (cut into chunks)

1 medium brown onion (diced)

1 teaspoon of garam masala

Salt and pepper (to taste)

2 cups of fish stock or preferably vegetable stock

1 medium brown onion (diced)

2 large zucchinis (chopped)

2 cloves garlic (crushed)

Directions:

1. First, you place all ingredients except the fish into a large pot over medium heat on the stove.
2. After which you bring the mixture to the boil, then lower the heat and allow to cook until the carrots have softened.
3. After that, you turn the heat down, add the fish and allow to cook for approximately 5 minutes, or until the fish flakes.
4. Then you serve immediately.

Gallbladder Cleansing Juice

Serves 1

4 beet leaves

½ lemon

1 medium beet (peeled)

1 stalk celery

2 red radishes

Directions:

First, you pass all ingredients through a juice extractor and drink.

Garlic Spicy Chicken

Serves 4

Ingredients

1 tablespoon of garlic powder

1 tablespoon of ground cumin

¼ cup of olive oil

3 pounds of chicken drumsticks

1 tablespoon of smoked paprika

½ teaspoon or preferably more of chili powder

½ teaspoon of salt

Directions:

1. First, you place all ingredients except chicken into a large bowl.
2. After which you add chicken drumsticks and coat them with the mixture well with your hands.
3. After that, you cook the chicken on a barbecue over medium heat for approximately 20 minutes on each side, or until cooked thoroughly.
4. Finally, you serve with a salad.

Sugar Free Coconut Balls

Ingredients

1 cup of unsweetened shredded coconut

Approximately ¼ cup of fresh lime juice

2 cups of raw cashews

2 tablespoons of coconut oil

Directions:

1. First, you place the cashews into a food processor and process until they become a fine meal.
2. After which you add all remaining ingredients and process until smooth.

NOTE: you may need a little more or better still a little less lime juice.

3. Remember, that this depends on how much moisture is present in the nuts and coconut you have purchased.
4. Finally, you shape the mixture into balls and store in an airtight container in the fridge.

Vegetarian Quinoa Pilaf

This recipe is low in fat, delicious, high protein, quick and easy to make.

Serves 4

Ingredients

2 cups of quinoa

1 medium red pepper (preferably capsicum), chopped

1 small head of broccoli (chopped)

2 large carrots (thinly sliced)

1 cup of diced pumpkin

1 tablespoon of dried oregano

Salt and pepper (to taste)

4 cups of vegetable stock

2 tablespoons of olive oil

1 medium yellow pepper (preferably capsicum) chopped

6 cherry tomatoes (halved)

2 medium zucchinis (chopped)

1 brown onion (chopped)

1 teaspoon of ground cumin

2 tablespoons of tomato paste

Directions:

1. First, you rinse the quinoa and cook it in a large pot in the vegetable stock for approximately 15 minutes, or until softened.
2. After which you heat the olive oil in a large pot over medium heat.
3. After that, you sauté the onion for approximately 3 minutes, or until softened.
4. Then you add all remaining ingredients except the quinoa.
5. At this point, you stir and cook gently until the vegetables have softened.

NOTE: you may need to add some water if the vegetables are sticking to the bottom of the pot.

6. Furthermore, once cooked, add vegetable mixture to the quinoa mixture.
7. Finally, you stir well and serve.

Tuna Steaks with Avocado

This recipe is a high protein, low carb meal that's delicious and helps you achieve your weight loss goals.

Serves 1

Ingredients

2 tablespoons of olive oil or ghee

2 tablespoons of lime juice

1 tuna steak

1 clove garlic (minced)

Salad ingredients

¼ red onion (sliced thinly)

Additional lime juice and olive oil (for dressing)

½ avocado (sliced)

2 large lettuce leaves (of your choice)

¼ cup of cherry tomatoes

Directions:

1. First, you place the oil, minced garlic and lime juice into a glass bowl.
2. After which you add the tuna steak and make sure it is well covered by the marinade.
3. After that, you cover the bowl and place in the fridge for about 2 hours.
4. Then you cook the tuna on a grill at medium heat, to your liking.
5. Finally, you arrange the tuna and salad on a plate and drizzle the salad with lime juice and olive oil.

Walnut Basil Pesto

This recipe is rich in antioxidants; this pesto is delicious served over chicken or fish.

Serves 4

Ingredients

½ cup of raw walnuts

¼ cup of fresh lime juice

¼ teaspoon of salt

3 cups of fresh basil leaves

½ cup of baby spinach leaves

½ teaspoon of grated lime zest

2 tablespoons of extra virgin olive oil or preferably macadamia nut oil

Directions:

1. First, you place all ingredients into a blender or food processor and blend until smooth.

Cumin Roasted Macadamia Nuts

This recipe is a deliciously indulgent snack that's high in heart-healthy monounsaturated fat.

Ingredients

½ teaspoon of smoked paprika

1 tablespoon of macadamia nut oil

2 cups of raw unsalted macadamia nuts

1 teaspoon of ground cumin

½ teaspoon of salt

Directions:

1. Meanwhile, you heat the oven to 355 degrees F.
2. After which you arrange the nuts on a lined baking tray and roast them for approximately 8 minutes, or until lightly golden.
3. Remember that the cooking time will depend on the size of the nuts.
4. Make sure you watch them carefully so they don't become too brown.
5. After that, you combine all remaining ingredients in a bowl.
6. Then you pour the hot nuts into the bowl, and cover them well with the oil and spice mixture.
7. At this point, you put the coated nuts back in the oven for up to 5 more minutes.
8. Finally, you serve nuts warm.

Garlic Bok Choy Stir Fry

Serves 2

Ingredients

2 cloves of garlic (minced)

1 tablespoon of coconut oil

4 bunches of bok choy (roughly chopped)

2 tablespoons of coconut aminos, or tamari, or soy sauce

Salt and pepper (to taste)

Directions:

1. First, you heat the coconut oil in a pan over medium heat.
2. After which you add the bok choy and stir.
3. After that, when it has wilted, add remaining ingredients.
4. Then you cook for an additional 2 minutes.
5. Finally, you serve with protein of your choice.

Easy Lemon Baked Salmon

This is a quick and easy low carb meal when you don't want to spend hours in the kitchen.

Serves 2

Ingredients

¼ cup of olive oil

1 teaspoon of ground cumin

Salt and pepper (to taste)

2 fresh salmon fillets

2 tablespoons of fresh lemon juice

2 tablespoons of finely chopped fresh dill

Directions:

1. First, you place all ingredients except salmon into a glass bowl and mix well.
2. After which you place the salmon fillets into the bowl and make sure they're well covered by the marinade.
3. After that, you cover the bowl and place in the fridge for two hours.
4. Then you bake the salmon in a preheated 400 degrees F oven for approximately 15 minutes, or until cooked to your liking.
5. Finally, you serve with a salad.

One Pan Chicken Dinner

Serves 4

Ingredients

1 head cauliflower (cut into florets)

2 carrots (sliced)

3 tablespoon of olive oil or preferably ghee

1 teaspoon of grated lemon zest

2 teaspoons of dried oregano

1-pound chicken thighs

½ cup of Kalamata olives (pitted)

1 brown onion (sliced)

¼ cup of fresh lemon juice

½ teaspoon of salt

Directions:

1. Meanwhile, you heat the oven to 400 degrees F.
2. After which you place chicken on a 7 x 11-inch baking dish.
3. After that, you arrange all other ingredients except lemon juice and olive oil on top of the chicken.

4. Then you drizzle with oil and juice and bake for approximately 50 minutes, or until the chicken is cooked through.

Low Carb Salmon Salad

Serves 1

Ingredients

3 cos lettuce leaves (chopped)

1 teaspoon of capers (sliced)

2 red radishes (sliced)

1 tablespoon of finely sliced fresh parsley

Lemon juice and olive oil (to taste)

6oz can salmon (drained)

1 boiled egg (sliced)

½ cup of cherry tomatoes (sliced in half)

½ small avocado (diced)

½ teaspoon of Dijon mustard

Directions:

1. First, you combine all ingredients in a bowl and serve.

Grilled Garlic Chicken

Serves 4

Ingredients

2 tablespoons of olive oil

4 garlic cloves (minced)

Salt and pepper (to taste)

2lbs chicken thighs

½ cup of balsamic vinegar

½ teaspoon of dried oregano

Directions:

1. First, you place all ingredients except chicken into a glass bowl.
2. After which you add chicken thighs and make sure they are all well covered by marinade.
3. After that, you cover the bowl and place in the fridge overnight.
4. Meanwhile, you heat the grill to medium heat.
5. Then you grill the chicken thighs for approximately 10 minutes on each side, or until cooked through.
6. Finally, you serve with a salad.

Detoxifying Green Smoothie

Serves 1

Ingredients

½ lime (peeled)

1 Lebanese cucumber

1 tablespoon of chia seeds

1 orange (peeled)

2 cups of baby spinach

1 cup of coconut milk

Directions:

1. First, you place all ingredients except chia seeds into a powerful blender and blend until smooth.
2. Then you stir in chia seeds and drink.

Garlic Roasted Broccoli

Make sure you serves 4 as a side dish

Ingredients

¼ cup of olive oil

Sea salt (to taste)

2 heads broccoli (chopped)

1 teaspoon of grated lemon zest

3 cloves garlic, crushed (it is optional)

Directions:

1. Meanwhile, you heat the oven to 320 degrees F.
2. After which you place the broccoli pieces on a greased oven tray.
3. After that, you combine all remaining ingredients and drizzle over broccoli.
4. Then you sprinkle with salt.
5. At this point, you roast in the oven for approximately 25 minutes, or until cooked to your liking.
6. Finally, you toss the broccoli around halfway through baking, to make sure it browns evenly.

Greek Yogurt and Cucumber Dip

It makes 3 cups of dip

Ingredients

1 peeled Lebanese cucumber

1 teaspoon of grated lime rind

1 clove garlic, crushed (it is optional)

2 cups of plain full fat Greek yogurt

2 tablespoons of fresh lime juice

1 tablespoon of finely chopped fresh dill

1 tablespoon of finely chopped fresh mint leaves

Directions:

1. First, you grate the cucumber finely in a medium sized bowl.
2. After which you add all remaining ingredients and mix well.
3. Then you cover the bowl and place in the fridge for 2 hours before serving.

Clean Green Smoothie

Serves 1

Ingredients

1 handful of baby spinach leaves

½ medium zucchini

1 cup of hemp milk

1 Lebanese cucumber

1 banana

1 tablespoon of coconut oil

2 tablespoons of hemp seeds

Directions:

First, you place all ingredients into a powerful blender and blend until smooth.

Grain and Dairy Free Almond Breakfast Pancakes

Serves 2

Ingredients

½ teaspoon of baking soda

¼ cup of almond or coconut milk

A few drops of liquid stevia (it is optional)

1 ½ cups of almond flour

3 large eggs (lightly whisked)

2 tablespoons of melted coconut oil

1 teaspoon of vanilla extract

Directions:

1. First, you place all ingredients into a blender and blend for one minute, or until well combined. NOTE: the batter will be quite thick.
2. After which you melt some coconut oil on a griddle at medium heat.
3. After that, you place heaped tablespoons of batter onto the griddle.

NOTE: these pancakes are easiest to cook if you make them little.

4. Then you cook each pancake for a few minutes and then flip over.
5. Make sure you serve with fruit.

Grain Free Bircher-Style Muesli

Serves 1

Ingredients

1 teaspoon of lime juice

2 tablespoons of chopped pecans

2 tablespoons of unsweetened shredded coconut

½ cup of milk of your choice

1 red unpeeled apple (coarsely grated)

1 tablespoon of chia seeds

2 tablespoons of flaked almonds

1 tablespoon of hemp seeds

A pinch of cinnamon and preferably clove powder

Directions:

1. First, you mix all ingredients together well and place in an airtight container.
2. After which you leave in the fridge overnight.
3. Then next morning you top with fruit of your choice and enjoy.

Creamy Cantaloupe Smoothie

Serves 1

Ingredients

½ cup of water

2 tablespoons of chia seeds

½ cup of full fat, canned coconut milk

1 cup of diced cantaloupe

2 tablespoons of whey protein powder

Directions:

First, you place all ingredients into a blender and blend until smooth.

Nut Free Bliss Balls

Ingredients

½ cup of dried apricots

½ cup of pumpkin seeds

½ cup of sunflower seeds

¼ teaspoon of ground nutmeg

6 medjool dates

¼ cup of raisins

1/3 cup of hemp seeds

½ teaspoon of ground cinnamon

Directions:

1. First, you place all ingredients into a food processor and process until smooth and the mixture comes together.
2. Then you shape the mixture into balls and keep in an airtight container in the fridge.

Dairy Free Creamy Lemon Sauce

Ingredients

1 small brown onion (very finely diced)

1 ½ tablespoons of lemon juice

2 tablespoons of olive oil

3/4 cup of full fat canned coconut cream

1/3 teaspoon of salt

Directions:

1. First, you heat the olive oil over medium heat in a saucepan
2. After which you add the onion and salt and cook gently just until it softens.
3. After that, you add coconut cream, stir and allow to simmer for up to 10 minutes, until the sauce thickens
4. Then you stir in lemon juice and take it off the heat
5. Finally, you serve.

Refreshing Watermelon Smoothie

Serves 1

Ingredients

Juice from ½ a lime

½ cup of nut or preferably hemp milk

1 cup of fresh watermelon cubes

1 tablespoon of chia seeds

A chopped, frozen banana

Directions:

First, you place all ingredients into a blender and blend until smooth.

Date and Tahini Fudge

This recipe is high in protein and minerals, nourishing your body and pleasing your taste buds.

Ingredients

½ cup of tahini

Approximately 1-2 tablespoons of almond meal

1 cup of fresh Medjool dates (pitted)

2 tablespoons of coconut oil

Directions:

1. First, you place all ingredients except almond meal in a food processor and process until well combined and smooth.
2. After which you remove mixture and place into a bowl.
3. After that, you add enough almond meal to reduce stickiness of the mixture.

NOTE: that the texture will depend on how much moisture is present in the dates and how oily the tahini is.

4. Then you spoon mixture into a square container and place in the freezer.

5. Finally, you cut into slices and serve.

Balsamic Roasted Tomatoes

This recipe is a powerful antioxidant that helps protect the prostate gland.

Make sure you serve 3 as a side dish

Ingredients

2 cloves garlic, crushed (it is optional)

3 tablespoons of olive oil

6 large, well ripened tomatoes (cut into chunks)

2 tablespoons of balsamic vinegar

Directions:

1. Meanwhile, you heat the oven to 320 degrees F.
2. After which you place the tomatoes on a lined oven tray and arrange the crushed garlic on top.
3. Then you drizzle with oil and vinegar and roast for approximately an hour.

Tender Grilled Baby Octopus

Serves 4

Ingredients

½ cup of olive oil

1 teaspoon of freshly grated lemon or better still lime zest

½ teaspoon of salt

2 pounds of baby octopus

¼ cup of lemon or preferably lime juice

2 cloves garlic (crushed)

Directions:

1. First, you clean and trim the baby octopus.
2. After which you bring 5 cups of water to the boil in a large pot.
3. After that, you turn the heat off and put the octopuses into the pot.
4. At this point, you leave them for one minute, then drain them and rinse under cold water.
5. Then you mix all remaining ingredients together in a glass bowl.
6. Furthermore, you add the octopuses, making sure they are well covered.

7. After which you cover the bowl and leave in the fridge for approximately 6 hours.
8. Meanwhile, you heat a grill on medium heat.
9. Finally, you grill the octopus for approximately 5 minutes.
10. Make sure you serve with a salad.

Mediterranean Beef Skewers

This recipe is a simple and delicious low carb meal when served with a salad or cooked vegetables.

Serves 4

Ingredients

1 red pepper (preferably capsicum), diced

1 tablespoon of dried oregano

1 teaspoon of dried marjoram

2 tablespoons of fresh lemon or preferably lime juice

2 lbs. of diced beef

2 cloves garlic (crushed)

1 teaspoon of dried thyme

4 tablespoons of olive oil

Skewers

Directions:

1. First, you combine all ingredients except the beef and red pepper in a glass bowl.

2. After which you add the beef, mix well, making sure it is all well covered by the marinade.
3. After that, you cover the bowl and place in the fridge overnight.
4. Meanwhile, you heat the grill to medium.
5. Then you thread the beef and pepper onto the skewers and cook for approximately 8 minutes, or until done to your liking.

Chicken and Orange Salad

This recipe is about to makes a quick and delicious weekday lunch, using pre-cooked chicken.

Serves 4

Ingredients

Meat from 1 cooked chicken

4 handfuls lettuce of your choice

2 large ripe tomatoes (chopped)

2 tablespoons of olive oil

2 oranges (peeled and sliced)

¼ cup of black olives (optional)

2 stalks celery (sliced)

1 Lebanese cucumber (sliced)

¼ cup of fresh lemon juice

Directions:

1. First, you place all salad ingredients into a large bowl
2. After which you drizzle with lemon juice and olive oil and toss
3. Then you serve

Sugar Free Banana Oat Bars

Makes about 8 squares

Ingredients

2 large, overly ripe bananas (mashed well)

2 tablespoons of goji berries

2 cups of rolled oats

1 teaspoon of vanilla extract

¼ cup of chopped toasted pecans

Directions:

1. **Meanwhile, you** heat the oven to 350 degrees F.
2. After which you line a 9 x 9-inch baking dish.
3. After that, you mix all ingredients extremely well in a bowl.
4. Then you pour into baking dish and bake for approximately 30 minutes, or until lightly browned.

Choc Mint Protein Smoothie

Serves 1

Ingredients

3 tablespoons of whey protein powder

1 tablespoon of chia seeds

1 ½ cups of milk of your choice (e.g. Almond or preferably cashew milk)

1 tablespoon of cacao or preferably cocoa powder

1 drop of peppermint essential oil

Directions:

First, you place all ingredients into a blender and blend until smooth.

Pumpkin and Pecan Casserole

This recipe is a healthy side dish when served with poultry or seafood.

Serves 4

Ingredients

3 cups of mashed roast sweet potato

1 tablespoon of maple syrup

2 cups of mashed roast pumpkin

2 eggs (whisked)

2 tablespoons of liquid coconut oil or ghee

Topping Ingredients

1 tablespoon of melted coconut oil or preferably ghee

1 teaspoon of pumpkin pie spice

1 cup of chopped pecans

1 teaspoon of maple syrup

Directions:

1. Meanwhile, you heat the oven to 350 degrees F.

2. After which you mix the casserole ingredients together well and place into a greased casserole dish.
3. After that, you mix all the topping ingredients together and sprinkle over casserole.
4. Then you bake for approximately 30 minutes, or until lightly browned.
5. Serve.

Kidney Cleansing Juice

Remember that the kidney-cleansing juice will provide your body with an extra cleansing boost.

Ingredients

1 large handful parsley

6 lettuce leaves

2 stalks of cclcry

1 orange (peeled)

1 Lebanese cucumber

Directions:

First, you pass all ingredients through a juice extractor and drink.

Chunky Avocado Salsa

I urge you to try this delicious Chunky Avocado Salsa as a side dish for any meal you see fit for the flavors.

Serves 2

Ingredients

1 large very ripe tomato (diced)

2 tablespoons of cilantro leave (chopped)

Salt and pepper (to taste)

1 large avocado (diced)

½ spring onion (finely diced)

2 tablespoons of lime juice

1 tablespoon of avocado oil or preferably macadamia nut oil

Directions:

1. First, you combine all ingredients in a bowl and toss gently.
2. Serve.

Conclusion

Ask yourself for a moment, if you could focus on one aspect of your well-being to transform all the others--and at the same time prevent health problems you didn't even know were lurking beneath the surface?

CPSIA information can be obtained
at www.ICGtesting.com
Printed in the USA
BVHW041956110620
581314BV00010B/605